Secret Cures For Asthma
and Heartburn

Secret Cures For Asthma and Heartburn

James Gordon Vatcher, MD

Library of Congress Control Number: 2011905414
ISBN: Hardcover   978-1-4628-5208-6
               Softcover   978-1-4628-5207-9
               Ebook   978-1-4628-5209-3

This book was printed in the United States of America.

To order additional copies of this book, contact:
Xlibris Corporation
1-888-795-4274
www.Xlibris.com
Orders@Xlibris.com
90848

Water, pure, liquid water, is the absolute necessity for any and all life on earth. It is ubiquitous, all around us, and within us as the major component of all our living cells. Most of the biomass on earth lives in water, whether in oceans, streams, lakes, rivers, etc. The forms that have migrated to live outside of the water, still require pure, liquid water for the conduct of the reactions of the living state, i.e. to be *"alive." All of their cells require water to function.*

Earth is called the "water planet" to differentiate it from the others, most of which are gases, except for the inner planets that are solid. Earth is largely solid except for the water. Earth has unique conditions that allow water to remain present in all of its forms; as a gas (steam), as a liquid, and as a solid (ice). The liquid form is the only one which supports, or is necessary, for the living state.

Water is so much a part of everything, so common all around us, that it has been "overlooked" or relatively ignored, until an unusual set of circumstances at the end of the last century brought it to the attention of Dr. Fereydoon Batmanghelidj. He was an Iranian M.D. who had been trained in London and had returned to his native Iran to set up some clinics for the care of the general population. His return came at the time that an Islamic Theocracy had set up a dictatorship and was executing the enemies of the state, one of which was Dr. Batmanghelidj. Instead of shooting him, he was given the job of caring for other prisoners, who were in similar situations. Almost all suffered from abdominal pain suggesting ulcer pain from stress gastritis. One evening, while he was walking in the hall of the prison, he was attracted by the screams and moans of one prisoner. He found this person curled up in a "fetal" position barely conscious and moaning with severe abdominal pain. The man had a known peptic ulcer and had been treating prior to incarceration with a common ulcer medication. He had used this already without any help.

Dr. Batmanghelidj had no medicine but told the suffering man to drink a glass of water because this was the medicine he had in the prison. He watched a few minutes and the man's pain seemed a little relieved. He told the prisoner to drink another glass of water and left to see someone else. When he returned a few minutes later, the man had improved even more. After another 2 glasses of water, the man seemed to be completely relieved, was sitting up and talking to friends who were amazed, surprised and happy to see his recovery.

Instead of assuming that the man was simply feigning his illness and recovery, Dr. Batmanghelidj wondered whether the water had actually been the "medicine" that effected the recovery, and he continued to treat others (several thousand), with similar abdominal pain, with water and observed their benefits. He wrote a paper about this effect of water on "heart burn" or ulcer disease while a prisoner. Upon his release, he came to the US and published more papers about this "discovery." He had found that humans lose the sensation of "thirst" early in life, but do not lose their need for water. The "thirst" simply is translated into some of the diseases we have as the result of becoming dehydrated. One of the most common of these is "heart burn."

We all like to solve problems, for ourselves, but also for others. If we are Dr.s, learned people, we like to be thought of as capable of solving problems for others. So with the problem of "heartburn." We know that acid is used, needed, for the digestion of organic material. It is produced in the gut; has been for ages. Why then has it begun to give pain then, relatively recently? How has the tissue of the gut been able to protect itself in the past, and what has happened to this protection now?

Of course, in solving the problem of "heartburn," the most obvious solution would be in counteracting the action of the acid. And so in the case of the present threat by the digesting acid, antacids seem to be the most obvious solution. Therefore we have used Sodium bicarbonate successfully. Unfortunately, some solutions have concomitant results that are harmful, and, so, with the case of bicarbonate of soda, the sodium was hard on the rest of the body, and contributed to increased incidence of heart failure.

The correction of this problem did not lead to a better understanding of the problem, but to a modification of the solution; ant-acids with less Sodium, and, therefore, we have "Tums" and "Roll-aids" etc. These sold, and sell, millions of dollars worth of medicines.

The next step would be to interrupt the production of the acid and we get the next generation of "antacids" the drugs that inhibit the actual production of the acid. These work very well, after a delay, and have become a modern drug of choice. However, as with all other misdirected solutions, these drugs have undesirable side effects that are becoming more obvious as time progresses.

A much better approach would be to think about what has protected the lining of the gut from the acid for all of these previous millennia. The lining of the gut, the stomach, is protected by a mucoid layer and mucus in more than 90% WATER. When we are dehydrated, this mucus layer becomes deficient and acid is allowed to reach the sensitive tissue of the gut wall and pain is produced. The most obvious solution therefore is to restore adequate hydration, that is to ingest more water. Water is the best, the cheapest, the most available and the most satisfactory solution to the problem of "heartburn" but it cannot be patented and therefore will remain a "secret" to the uninformed. It is less handy than a simple tablet, though with the availability of water bottles, this "availability" and simplicity is less so.

As human beings, we look for the quick solution and don't think so much about the long term effects until troubled by them. So, in the case of water curing heartburn, we don't think in terms of water possibly not only curing heartburn, but also preventing this by keeping the body hydrated and maintaining the mucoid layer to prevent future trouble. The medical community is also not interested in curing the basic, underlying problem once it has solved the immediate one. The Dr. gets paid for treating the disease, not for curing the problem. In fact, if the problem were to be "cured" there would be no more people needing help or needing to pay for care.

Human beings are always on the lookout for the "easy" way of doing things, which may not always be the best or most natural way. In addition to the antacids we have first begun to use, we have more "refined" methods of overcoming the effects of acid on health, living organic tissue. We have the acid neutralizing drugs such as TUMS and Maalox. Next we have the drugs that slow down the production of the acid, Zantac and Tagamet that block the Histamine (more about this later) receptors and slow the production of the acid.

Here again we have the usual human attempt to solve a "problem," that is, getting rid of what is thought to be the problem, by counteracting or reducing the offending agent, the acid. There is no attempt to investigate to see how nature may by already been solving this problem, just go right to the agent itself, the acid. The idea that the body may have already solved the problem by the formation of a mucoid layer does not enter into the thinking of those who feel they have been called upon to solve a problem caused by the presence of a "normal" substance (a substance used by the body to digest food, which has been around for millennia and will be around as long as people eat, and need to digest food for energy, etc.).

This solution has been overlooked for generations, and it is "Water." "Water" is the "miracle cure" for "heart-burn. Water increases the mucoid layer protecting the lining of the gut against the action of the acid. The next question is just how much water is needed to attain and maintain adequate hydration. This is simple and depends upon the size of the individual. The formula is one ounce of water for every two pounds body weight. If you take one half of your body weight, in pounds, then that is the number of ounces of water to take in a day.

This means just water, not tea, or coffee, or some other fluid. These are alright to use but must not be counted as part of the daily needed intake of WATER. Many fluids can be actually dehydrating, liquids such as alcohol, wine, beer, etc., are dehydrating and must not be considered as part of the body's need for water, in fact should be a sign to increase the actual water intake. Juices, such as orange juice or other fruit juice, are tasty, and not to be shunned, just not to be considered as part of the needed one ounce of water per 2 pounds of body weight. Orange juice is high in Potassium and a tendency to take a large amount with the thought that it is "healthy" can be unhealthy.

In addition to water, salt in small amounts is a necessity. Take about a quarter teaspoonful for every quart of water (32 ounces). This is in the face of popular medical advice to restrict salt. It is possible to get sick from taking too much salt, just as it is possible to get sick from "too" much water. This is the meaning of the words "too much." But the limitation noted will provide enough sodium (salt) without overloading the system.

Caffeine is also slightly dehydrating, and care must be taken to limit the use of this important chemical. Not to eliminate it entirely, but to recognize that it may increase the body's need for water.

In the case of Asthma, here again we see a problem resulting from the response of the body to dehydration. We lose about

1 quart of water from the lungs when we exhale or breathe out. This is the "steam" we see when breathing in cold weather. In order to reduce this, the body constricts the small tubes carrying the air from the lungs to the outside. This constriction produces an audible "wheeze" at the end of expiration in those who are afflicted with this problem. Not everyone is troubled by this problem, just as we are all individuals and each of us reacts to the world around us in different ways.

In the asthmatic, this constriction obstructs the outflow of air thus hampering breathing in a special way. The medical world has developed several means for resolving this problem and these are the various treatments to which the asthmatic is exposed. The substance causing the constriction, trying to prevent the loss of water from the lungs, is called Histamine. This is a very useful chemical with many other functions, but the asthmatic is particularly sensitive to the effect in the lungs. Histamine is a drought management chemical, serving to prevent the loss of water from a marginally dehydrated individual, someone who has become dehydrated through failing to take in adequate amounts of water over several days, weeks, months, years.

Anti-histamines are one means of counteracting the histamine effect, just as antacids are in the case of heartburn. There are also bronco-dilators that work to open up the bronchioles that carry the air out of the lungs (along with the water-vapor). Since Histamine is involved in what are called "allergic" reactions, Corticosteroids are also used with some benefit.

Nothing works perfectly, or forever, so we have many different treatment regimens all of which seem to work for a time then must be changed, or altered. As individuals, we have varying responses to those conditions that cause us to wheeze and therefore varying responses to the treatments. Sometimes more intensive treatment is needed than at others and IV administration of the various drugs is required as well as hospitalization for the administration of Oxygen to maintain life. Even with the best and most intensive treatments, many people die each year from the complications of Asthma.

Of course, the Medical Care Industry embraces the idea that Asthma is incurable. This means there is a vast reservoir of people who will be chronically ill and in need of treatment for most of their lives. While the members of the Medical Care Industry like to think that they are interested in the welfare of others, they are human beings and have varying degrees of self-interest. The members of the Medical Care Industry are experts in developing exciting, stimulating, complicated new therapies, tests, insights, medicines, etc., in the nature of this incurable affliction, and they are handsomely rewarded for these efforts, and many are looked-up-to as benefactors. To find a cure is unthinkable, and counterproductive.

The Asthma and Allergy Foundation of America notes that 40,000 people miss school or work every day due to Asthma, and that 30,000 people have Asthma attacks per day. Also of note is that 5,000 people visit Emergency Rooms every day, for treatment of their Asthma, and that 1,000 people are hospitalized in any day because of their Asthma needing extra care. In addition, 11 people die every day from their Asthma.

There are 60 million people with this disease, this "incurable" disease, costing 18 Million Dollars a year for their care. Of course this cost is not "lost." It provides the income of the Medical Care Industry practitioners, hospital workers, emergency room personnel, etc., and is taxable by the government, so "we" all profit from the disease, discomfort, of those few unfortunates who have Asthma (or Allergies). The only sufferers are those with this disease. They are interested in a "Cure" but they are powerless individuals who are ignorant and only selfishly interested in their own welfare.

This is most unfortunate since it is totally preventable when the underlying problem of dehydration is recognized and corrected. While the role of water in the prevention of Histamine release has not been proven, it has been suggested. No institution will undertake the necessary studies, but an individual can do this. Taking a little (or a lot) of water a day would not be expensive, not be toxic and in a few days a benefit could be noted.

Water has been proposed as a prime antihistamine, one that is inexpensive, non-toxic and readily available. In some marine animals, while the stress of dehydration seems to cause the increased production and release of Histamine, this has not been proven in mammals. In science, we seem to stress the need for a positive "proof" before we can do something. The value of a negative proof is of equal importance, and may be more valuable when a positive proof is impractical.

With all of the money and effort that have been put forth in the study of antihistamines, it was totally accidental that no one, other than Dr. Batmanghelidj, would be championing the use of water as an antihistamine in the treatment of Asthma, and other diseases. Except that there is no money in "Water." Millions of people suffer from Asthma, and thousands die as the result of this disease, but little attention is given to water as a preventative. At the same time, much attention is given to the use of antihistamines, the agents which counteract the actions of Histamine.

The establishment of proper hydration reduces the amount of Histamine the body produces and therefore the amount of constriction of the bronchioles. Asthma, which I was taught to consider incurable, is totally curable, really preventable, by the proper ingestion of adequate amounts of simple water.

There is so much money involved in the treatments of Asthma, and heartburn, and all of the other "diseases" that can be removed by the simple hydration of all of us, that this is an imposing superstructure and will mean that hydration will remain a secret. This will remain a secret except to those involved and seriously ill with the problem, and for whom the other treatments have proven unsuccessful. I feel hopeless in making these observations, like the little boy who observed that the emperor was really wearing no clothes, while all of the others seemed not to want to notice this (obvious) lack.

The present medical organization allows for, even encourages over specialization, and over super-specialization. Disease is the condition that brings the patient to the attention of the medical community and thus is the (obvious) first focus of attention by the Dr.s. As human beings we tend to focus on what is in front of us, and, therefore, to study and learn more about this. In a sense, this leaves us blind to what else is around us, and also blind to this blindness.

There is simply more money, and less time involved, for the specialist in limiting his or her field of concern since there is less time needed to give the appearance of expertise in a limited field of study. One can learn the language of a smaller field and appear to be more expert to colleagues (those who appoint people to faculty positions) whereas treating real people, real patients, is time-consuming, complicated and frustrating and doesn't yield pleasant, recordable results.

Of course treating real patients would require some attention being given to an individual patient, something that is fraught with sloppiness and possible error. Because of this, the individual patient finds a hard time in locating a "Dr." who has specialized in his or her particular malady. This leads to the bouncing around of patients until the patient reaches the "right" specialist or gets well without further help. The patient exists for the welfare of the medical establishment, rather than the other way around. Disease is the condition that brings the patient to the attention of the medical establishment and this becomes their focus of attention. This is very natural, but it completely ignores the fact that it is the "patient" that brings the "disease" to the attention of the Dr.

Of course studying the whole patient is nearly impossible, because of the complexity of each individual. This is where, and why, the work of Dr. Batmanghelidj becomes important. Each of us needs WATER, and each of us tends to become deficient in this material. Simply advising each person to become hydrated is good advice and will solve many of mankind's problems. The universal advice that reduces the complexity of mankind to a small degree.

While studying the disease, or anatomy, seems to reduce the complexity of the *problem of providing medical advice, it simply spreads it out and leaves the individual without an advisor. The medical person can advise the patient's "heart" or "pancreas" but not the whole patient.*

This gives rise to the basic misunderstanding that plagues "medicine" today. The business of the Medical Care Industry is the treatment of diseases. It is the "treatment" of diseases, though this would seem to be a part of, a concomitant of, the treatment of disease. The Medial Care Industry has been able to sell its services by calling them "Health Care" but they are only different forms of Medical Care. Diagnostic tests, studies, operations, etc., are all expensive, ingenious, approaches to the study and treatment of disease, but they are no different from the processes and procedures that preceded them. Cures occur in the cases of the treatment of broken bones, or tying off of a torn splenic pedicle artery, but, in the majority of the "diseases" which we have described today, "diagnosed" today, there is only "treatment." Hypertension, hypercholesterolemia, asthma, allergies, some forms of diabetes mellitus, heartburn, etc. all have treatments, but no present "cure." These have no "cures" and only need a life-long investment in their treatment.

This fundamental dissonance, misunderstanding, of what we seek when we seek medical care, the usual medical care, weighs on the minds of both patients and practitioners. It may contribute to the frequency of suicides and early deaths among practitioners. The basic BUSINESS of the Medical Care Industry is the TREATMENT of chronic disease and not its cure. The patient wants cure.

The public has been sold Medical Care by calling it "Health Care." It does this without a good definition for "Health" and no one has really been thinking about this to notice the discrepancy. Simply put, we now define Health in terms of disease. If you are not sick then you are healthy. There are other more "profound" and meaningless, high sounding definitions but it boils down to something to do with absence of illness. This means you must have a defined (approved) disease that has been treated, meaning you need the Medical Care Industry personage to define, diagnose, a disease, meaning health is based on a Medical Care Diagnosis.

What is needed is a definition of "health" that is not related to sickness, is not related to Medical Care. One such could be in terms of Energy. A person is "healthy" when he or she has enough Energy to do the things they feel they want and or need to do. With the idea of Energy in relation to "Health" we can treat those cases in *which there is no clear cut diagnosis of specific disease needing specific treatment, which is most of the time. Application or introduction of Energy can be afforded to anybody, will do no harm, and may be beneficial.*

President Andrew Jackson is an example of a man who might have been considered seriously ill, but he had enough Energy to accomplish what he felt he needed to do, so how does he fit the definition. He had terminal heart and kidney disease, but mentally felt it necessary to continue to exercise his presidential powers to achieve his goals. His diseases, which would have totally incapacitated lesser men, did not deprive him of the Energy he needed to function as President. In this real sense, he was "healthy." Obviously the definition is not exact. Many "healthy" people may have as yet undiagnosed cancers, etc.

Such ideas have been around along with traditional treatments, since the traditional treatments have not seemed to be as effective as their proponents have wished. These have been referred to as alternative medicine, or holistic or other treatments and indicate our desire to find something that will work better than traditional care. (One of the admonitions given to physicians for making money is to "use mankind's ills." (A variation of this is to use mankind ill.))

Many of these techniques have been used for millennia. Heat, in the form of saunas, is time-honored, and is be available now in the form of far-infra-red lamps for relatively small amounts of money. Water of course is the first "treatment" to be considered. Vitamin C in therapeutic doses of 5 to 10 Grams a day, or more, to tolerance is again benign and must be considered. Ultra-violet irradiation of blood is another benign treatment with great value and kills many of the more worrisome infections that occur nowadays. Things like MRSA bacteria, the AIDS virus, almost any and all infections, etc. There are many more benign therapies, of which these are only a few. More may be proposed by the many who want to jump on the bandwagon and make money by advertising their particular wares. The one value of having approved diagnoses is that it puts some limit on what can be marketed as a therapy. The bad part of this, our present plan, is that there is no way to prevent the distortions that human beings can bring to any system when not guided by some common sense of what is the real, basic purpose of the whole program.

Language can be used to justify any distortion. It is the job of thinking people to separate the parts of the language that represent science and what parts represent insanity. The present misrepresentation of Medical Care as Health Care is an insanity that will eventually become obvious, after trillions have been spent and people have been involved in heated arguments over what is and what is not important. Many will have suffered and died because of the humanness, and self-serving, blind "conservatism" of the medical establishment that seeks to justify the do-nothing "status-quo" as being in the best interests of safe patient care. Vitamin C effectively kills cancer cells without harming normal cells, ultraviolet-light kills many pathogens, silver is an excellent antibiotic, DMSO is a potent natural healing chemical and so on. None of these can be used because of Medical Care Industry prohibitions, or blind obstruction.

Of course, there is always hope, but this must be combined with the efforts of those imperfect individuals like ourselves who think they see solutions that are different and not self-limited.

ETC.